The Happy Pregnancy Handbook

A Guide to Enjoying Your Pregnancy
Journey

Lori N. Martin

Table Of Content

Conclusion

Appendix

Introduction

Welcome to one of the most exciting journeys of your life! Your pregnancy journey is a unique and transformative experience that will change you in ways you never thought possible. From the moment you discover that you're pregnant, your life will be filled with wonder, excitement, and joy.

But pregnancy can also be a time of uncertainty and anxiety. You might be wondering what changes to expect in your body, how to manage common pregnancy symptoms, and how to prepare for labor and delivery. You may also be feeling overwhelmed by the sheer amount of information available online and from well-meaning friends and family members.

That's where "The Happy Pregnancy Handbook" comes in. We've created this guide to help you navigate the ups and downs of pregnancy with ease, providing you with the information, tools, and resources you need to enjoy a happy, healthy pregnancy.

Throughout this book, we'll take you through each stage of your pregnancy journey, from the early weeks of your pregnancy to the postpartum period. We'll cover everything from prenatal care to preparing for labor and delivery, and from breastfeeding to caring for your newborn.

But we won't just focus on the physical aspects of pregnancy. We'll also help you cultivate a positive mindset and emotional well-being throughout your pregnancy, helping you find inner peace, mindfulness, and joy.

So, whether you're a first-time mom or an experienced parent, we invite you to embark on this journey with us. Let's explore the wonders of pregnancy together and help you create a happy, healthy, and fulfilling pregnancy journey.

Preparing for Pregnancy

Before you embark on your pregnancy journey, it's important to take some time to prepare your body and mind. Preconception planning can help ensure that you have the healthiest possible pregnancy and that your baby gets the best possible start in life.

Here are some tips to help you prepare for pregnancy:

1. Schedule a preconception checkup: Before you start trying to conceive, it's a good idea to schedule a preconception checkup with your healthcare provider. This visit will help identify any health issues that might affect your pregnancy, such as diabetes or high blood pressure.

2. Start taking prenatal vitamins: Prenatal vitamins are an important part of preconception planning, as they contain the essential nutrients that your baby

needs to grow and develop. Make sure to choose a prenatal vitamin that contains folic acid, which can help prevent birth defects.

3. Get to a healthy weight: Being underweight or overweight can affect your fertility and your pregnancy. Try to get to a healthy weight before you start trying to conceive.

4. Quit smoking and avoid alcohol: Smoking and alcohol can both have negative effects on fertility and pregnancy. If you smoke, quit before you start trying to conceive. And if you drink alcohol, stop or cut back to no more than one drink per day.

5. Eat a healthy diet: A healthy diet can help support fertility and a healthy pregnancy. Focus on eating a variety of fruits, vegetables, whole grains, lean protein, and healthy fats.

6. Familiarize yourself with your menstrual cycle and ovulation. This can help you identify your most fertile days and increase your chances of conceiving.

7. Consider genetic counseling if you have a family history of genetic disorders. This can help you understand your risk of passing on genetic conditions to your child and explore options for prenatal testing.

By taking these steps to prepare for pregnancy, you'll be setting yourself up for a healthy, happy pregnancy journey.

Part I: Pregnancy Basics

Chapter 1: Understanding Pregnancy

Understanding pregnancy is an important part of preparing for your journey. Pregnancy is a complex process that involves many changes in your body and your life. Here are some key things to know about pregnancy:

1. How pregnancy happens: Pregnancy occurs when a sperm fertilizes an egg and the fertilized egg implants in the uterus. This usually happens during ovulation, when an egg is released from the ovary and travels down the fallopian tube.

2. The stages of pregnancy: Pregnancy is divided into three trimesters, each lasting about 13 weeks. During the first trimester, your baby's organs and body systems begin to develop. During the second trimester, your baby grows and becomes more active. And during the third trimester, your baby prepares for birth by getting into position.

3. Common pregnancy symptoms: Many women experience common pregnancy symptoms such as morning sickness, fatigue, and mood changes. Other common symptoms include back pain, constipation, and frequent urination.

4. Prenatal care: Prenatal care is essential for a healthy pregnancy. This includes

regular checkups with your healthcare provider, prenatal testing, and monitoring your health and your baby's health.

5. Labor and delivery: Labor and delivery is the process of giving birth to your baby. This can be a long and intense process, but there are many ways to manage pain and cope with the challenges of childbirth.

6. Potential complications: While most pregnancies are healthy and uncomplicated, there are some potential complications that can occur. These can include gestational diabetes, preeclampsia, and preterm labor. It's important to be aware of the signs and

symptoms of these complications and to seek medical attention if necessary.

7. Emotional changes: Pregnancy can be a time of intense emotional changes, including excitement, anxiety, and mood swings. It's important to take care of your emotional well-being during pregnancy, which can include practicing self-care, seeking support from loved ones, and talking to a mental health professional if necessary.

8. Postpartum period: The postpartum period is the time after childbirth when your body and life adjust to having a new baby. This can be a challenging time, as you recover from childbirth and adjust to caring for a newborn. It's

important to have a support system in place during this time, which can include family and friends, healthcare providers, and postpartum support groups.

By understanding these key aspects of pregnancy, you'll be better equipped to navigate the challenges and joys of your pregnancy journey. Remember to take care of yourself and your baby, listen to your body, and seek medical attention if necessary. With the right preparation and support, you can have a healthy, happy pregnancy and a beautiful new addition to your family.

Chapter 2: Your Body During Pregnancy

During pregnancy, your body goes through many changes to support the growth and development of your baby. Here are some of the ways that your body changes during pregnancy:

1. Hormonal changes: During pregnancy, your body produces high levels of hormones, such as estrogen and progesterone, to support the growth of your baby. These hormones can cause many changes in your body, including fatigue, nausea, and breast tenderness.

2. Weight gain: During pregnancy, it's normal to gain weight as your baby grows. Most women will gain between 25 and 35 pounds during pregnancy, although the amount of weight gain can vary depending on your pre-pregnancy weight.

3. Changes in your uterus: Your uterus will grow significantly during pregnancy to accommodate your growing baby. This can cause discomfort and pressure in your abdomen.

4. Changes in your breasts: Your breasts will also undergo changes during pregnancy as they prepare for lactation. You may experience breast tenderness

and swelling, and your nipples may become more sensitive.

5. Changes in your skin: Many women experience changes in their skin during pregnancy, such as darkening of the areolas, stretch marks, and acne.

6. Changes in your cardiovascular system: Your cardiovascular system will undergo changes during pregnancy to support the increased blood flow and oxygen needed for your baby's growth. This can cause your heart rate and blood pressure to increase.

7. Changes in your digestive system: Pregnancy can also affect your digestive system, causing symptoms

such as constipation, heartburn, and nausea.

It's important to remember that every pregnancy is different, and you may experience some or all of these changes to varying degrees. If you have any concerns about the changes in your body during pregnancy, be sure to talk to your healthcare provider. They can provide guidance and support to help you have a healthy, comfortable pregnancy.

Chapter 3: Prenatal Care

Prenatal care is an essential part of a healthy pregnancy. Here are some key things to know about prenatal care:

1. The importance of early prenatal care: Early prenatal care is important for a healthy pregnancy. Your healthcare provider can perform important tests and screenings to monitor your health and the health of your baby, and can provide guidance and support throughout your pregnancy.

2. Prenatal appointments: During your prenatal appointments, your healthcare provider will monitor your health and

the health of your baby. This can include measuring your weight and blood pressure, listening to your baby's heartbeat, and performing ultrasounds and other tests as needed.

3. Prenatal testing: Prenatal testing can help detect potential health problems in you or your baby. This can include blood tests, ultrasounds, and other diagnostic tests. Your healthcare provider can help determine which tests are appropriate for you based on your individual health needs and risk factors.

4. Nutrition and exercise: Good nutrition and regular exercise are important for a healthy pregnancy. Your healthcare provider can provide guidance on a

healthy diet and safe exercise options during pregnancy.

5. Managing pregnancy symptoms: Many women experience common pregnancy symptoms such as morning sickness, fatigue, and mood changes. Your healthcare provider can provide guidance and support for managing these symptoms and ensuring your comfort and well-being.

6. Preparing for childbirth: Prenatal care can also include education and preparation for childbirth. This can include information on pain management options, childbirth classes, and creating a birth plan.

7. High-risk pregnancies: Some pregnancies may be considered high-risk due to factors such as advanced maternal age, pre-existing medical conditions, or a history of pregnancy complications. If you have a high-risk pregnancy, your healthcare provider may recommend additional monitoring and care to ensure the health and safety of you and your baby.

8. The role of partners and support persons: Partners and support persons can play an important role in prenatal care, childbirth, and postpartum recovery. Your healthcare provider can provide guidance on how partners and support persons can be involved in your care and provide emotional

support and practical assistance during this exciting and challenging time.

9. Postpartum care: Prenatal care also includes planning and preparing for postpartum care. This can include guidance on breastfeeding, managing postpartum symptoms, and monitoring for postpartum complications such as postpartum depression.

By prioritizing prenatal care and working closely with your healthcare provider, you can ensure a healthy pregnancy, a safe childbirth experience, and a smooth transition to postpartum life. Remember to communicate openly with your healthcare provider, seek support from loved ones, and prioritize self-care as you navigate this transformative and exciting time in your life.

Chapter 4: Nutrition and Exercise During Pregnancy

Nutrition and exercise are important components of a healthy pregnancy. Here are some key things to know about nutrition and exercise during pregnancy:

1. Nutritional needs: During pregnancy, your body has increased nutritional needs to support the growth and development of your baby. This includes a higher intake of calories, protein, and certain vitamins and minerals. Your healthcare provider can provide guidance on a healthy and balanced diet that meets your individual nutritional needs.

2. Food safety: It's important to practice safe food handling and preparation during pregnancy to reduce the risk of foodborne illness. This includes avoiding raw or undercooked meats, fish, and eggs, and washing fruits and vegetables thoroughly.

3. Hydration: Staying hydrated is important during pregnancy to support your overall health and the health of your baby. Aim to drink at least 8-10 cups of water per day, and more if you are exercising or in a hot climate.

4. Exercise: Regular exercise during pregnancy can help improve your physical and emotional well-being, and

may reduce the risk of certain pregnancy complications such as gestational diabetes and preeclampsia. Talk to your healthcare provider about safe and appropriate exercise options during pregnancy.

5. Pelvic floor exercises: Pelvic floor exercises, also known as Kegels, can help strengthen the muscles that support your bladder, uterus, and rectum. This can help reduce the risk of urinary incontinence and other pelvic floor problems during pregnancy and after childbirth.

6. Weight gain: It's important to gain weight at a healthy rate during pregnancy to support the growth and

development of your baby. Your healthcare provider can provide guidance on how much weight gain is appropriate for you based on your individual health needs and body mass index (BMI).

7. Special considerations: If you have pre-existing medical conditions, such as diabetes or high blood pressure, or if you are carrying multiples, your healthcare provider may recommend additional nutritional or exercise interventions to ensure the health and safety of you and your baby.

8. Emotional health: Good nutrition and exercise are important for both physical and emotional health during pregnancy.

However, it's also important to prioritize your emotional well-being by seeking support from loved ones, participating in stress-reducing activities such as yoga or meditation, and seeking professional help if needed.

9. Postpartum exercise: After giving birth, it's important to gradually return to exercise in a safe and appropriate manner. Your healthcare provider can provide guidance on when it's safe to resume exercise, what types of exercise are appropriate, and how to adjust your exercise routine as needed.

Remember, every pregnancy is unique, and what works for one person may not work for another. Talk to your healthcare provider about your individual nutrition and exercise needs during pregnancy, and listen to your body to ensure that you are staying healthy and feeling your best.

Chapter 5: Managing Common Pregnancy Symptoms

While pregnancy is an exciting and transformative time, it can also be accompanied by a range of uncomfortable symptoms. Here are some common pregnancy symptoms and tips for managing them:

1. Nausea and vomiting: Many women experience nausea and vomiting, especially during the first trimester. Eating small, frequent meals throughout the day, avoiding greasy or spicy foods, and staying hydrated can help reduce these symptoms.

2. Fatigue: Pregnancy can be tiring, especially during the first and third trimesters. Getting enough rest, napping when needed, and delegating tasks to loved ones can help manage fatigue.

3. Heartburn and indigestion: These symptoms can be caused by the hormonal changes of pregnancy and the pressure of the growing uterus on the stomach. Eating small, frequent meals, avoiding spicy or acidic foods, and propping yourself up with pillows while sleeping can help reduce these symptoms.

4. Constipation: Hormonal changes and the pressure of the growing uterus can

slow down the digestive system, leading to constipation. Eating a high-fiber diet, staying hydrated, and getting regular exercise can help alleviate this symptom.

5. Back pain: As your belly grows and your posture changes, back pain is a common pregnancy symptom. Gentle exercise, such as prenatal yoga or swimming, and wearing supportive shoes can help manage back pain.

6. Swelling: Swelling, especially in the feet and ankles, is common during pregnancy. Staying hydrated, elevating your feet, and wearing comfortable shoes can help reduce swelling.

7. Mood changes: Hormonal changes during pregnancy can lead to mood swings and feelings of anxiety or depression. Staying connected with loved ones, engaging in stress-reducing activities, and seeking professional help if needed can help manage these symptoms.

8. Braxton Hicks contractions: These are mild, painless contractions that can occur throughout pregnancy. To manage these, try changing positions, drinking water, and practicing relaxation techniques.

Remember, every pregnancy is unique, and what works for one person may not work for another. Talk to your healthcare provider about your individual symptoms and needs, and listen to your body to ensure that you are managing your symptoms and staying healthy during pregnancy.

Part II: Preparing for Labor and Delivery

Chapter 6: Stages of Labor

Labor is the process by which your body prepares for and gives birth to your baby. There are three stages of labor:

- First stage: This is the longest stage of labor, lasting from the onset of regular contractions to when the cervix is fully dilated (opened) to 10 centimeters. During this stage, contractions become longer, stronger, and more frequent, and your cervix will begin to efface (thin out) and dilate. This stage can last anywhere from a few hours to more than a day. During the first stage of labor, your healthcare provider will monitor your progress by checking your cervix for dilation and effacement. They may also monitor your baby's heart rate to ensure that they are tolerating the contractions well. As your contractions become stronger and more frequent, you may begin to feel discomfort or pain. There are various pain management techniques available, such as breathing exercises, relaxation techniques, massage, and medication. Your healthcare provider can discuss these options with you and help you decide which ones may work best for you.

- Second stage: This is the pushing stage, which begins when the cervix is fully dilated and ends with the birth of your baby. During this stage, you will push to help your baby move through the birth canal. Once you reach the second stage of labor, your healthcare provider will guide you through the pushing process. They may encourage you to try different positions, such as squatting, sitting, or lying on your side, to help your baby move through the birth canal. They will also monitor your baby's heart rate and may use tools such as forceps or a vacuum to assist with delivery if needed.

- Third stage: After your baby is born, you will enter the third stage of labor. Your healthcare provider will help deliver the placenta, which is the organ that nourished your baby during pregnancy. You may experience mild contractions or discomfort during this stage, but it usually lasts only a few minutes.

There are different ways to give birth, including vaginal birth and cesarean birth (C-section). Vaginal birth is the most common way to give birth and typically has a shorter recovery time. However, there are situations where a C-section may be necessary for the health and safety of you and your baby.

It's important to remember that every labor and delivery is unique, and your experience may not follow a typical progression. Be sure to talk to your healthcare provider about your individual needs and preferences for labor and delivery.

Chapter 7: Signs of Labor

As your due date approaches, you may be wondering how to tell when labor is starting. Here are some signs that labor may be near:

1. Contractions: These are the most common signs of labor. True labor contractions become stronger, longer, and more frequent over time. You may also feel them in your lower back or abdomen, and they may come and go in a regular pattern.

2. Water breaking: Your amniotic sac may rupture, causing fluid to leak from your vagina. This can happen before or during labor.

3. Cervical changes: Your cervix may start to dilate (open) and efface (thin out) in preparation for labor. Your healthcare provider can check your cervix during a prenatal exam to monitor these changes.

4. Backache: You may experience a dull ache or pressure in your lower back as your baby moves into position for birth.

5. Bloody show: This is a small amount of blood-tinged mucus that may be expelled from your vagina as your cervix starts to dilate.

6. Nesting instinct: Some women experience a burst of energy and an urge to clean or organize their home in the days leading up to labor.

It's important to note that not all women experience these signs of labor, and some women may experience false labor contractions or Braxton Hicks contractions that can be mistaken for labor. If you are unsure whether you are experiencing true labor, contact your healthcare provider. They can help determine if it's time to go to the hospital or birthing center. It's also important to keep in mind that not all women experience these signs before labor starts, and some signs may occur without leading to labor. If you are unsure if you are in labor, contact your healthcare provider for guidance. They can help you determine if it's time to go to the hospital or birthing center.

Chapter 8: Pain Management Options

Labor and delivery can be a challenging and sometimes painful experience. Fortunately, there are various pain management options available to help make the process more manageable. Here are some common pain management options for labor and delivery:

1. Breathing techniques: Focusing on deep breathing and relaxation can help you cope with the pain of contractions.

2. Massage: Gentle massage from your partner, doula, or healthcare provider can help you relax and ease tension during labor.

3. Hydrotherapy: Taking a warm bath or shower can help ease muscle tension and provide pain relief.

4. Medication: There are various medications available to help manage pain during labor and delivery. Some common options include opioids, epidural anesthesia, and nitrous oxide.

5. Positioning: Changing positions, such as squatting, kneeling, or standing, can help your baby move through the birth canal and relieve pain.

6. Acupuncture or acupressure: These techniques involve placing needles or

pressure on specific points of the body to promote relaxation and pain relief.

7. Relaxation techniques: These may include visualization, meditation, or listening to calming music. They can help you stay focused and reduce anxiety.

It's important to discuss your pain management options with your healthcare provider before labor and delivery, so you can make an informed decision about which options may work best for you. Keep in mind that every woman's labor and delivery experience is unique, and what works for one woman may not work for another.

Chapter 9: Birth Plans

A birth plan is a document that outlines your preferences and goals for labor and delivery. While it's important to keep in mind that unexpected situations may arise during childbirth, having a birth plan can help you communicate your wishes to your healthcare provider and support team. Here are some things to consider when creating a birth plan:

1. Location of birth: Do you plan to give birth in a hospital, birthing center, or at home?

2. Support team: Who do you want present during labor and delivery? This

may include a partner, family members, or a doula.

3. Pain management: What pain management options do you prefer? Do you want to try natural methods, or do you want to have access to medications or an epidural?

4. Monitoring and interventions: Do you have preferences for fetal monitoring, such as intermittent monitoring or continuous monitoring? What are your preferences for interventions such as artificial rupture of membranes, induction, or assisted delivery (such as forceps or vacuum)?

5. Positioning: Do you have preferences for positions during labor and delivery, such as standing, sitting, or using a birthing ball or stool?

6. Feeding preferences: Do you plan to breastfeed or bottle-feed? Do you have any special requests or preferences for how your baby is fed after delivery?

7. Newborn care: Do you have any preferences for your baby's care immediately after birth, such as delayed cord clamping, skin-to-skin contact, or routine procedures like Vitamin K injection or eye ointment?

8. Special considerations: If you have any medical conditions or complications

during pregnancy, you may need to include special considerations in your birth plan. For example, if you have gestational diabetes, you may need to monitor your blood sugar during labor.

9. Communication preferences: How do you prefer to communicate with your healthcare provider and support team during labor and delivery? Do you have any special requests for how information is shared with you?

Remember that a birth plan is a personal document, and there is no one "right" way to create one. Your birth plan should reflect your individual preferences, values, and goals. Be sure to discuss your birth plan with your healthcare provider and support team, and remember that it's okay to change your mind or make adjustments during labor and delivery. The most important thing is to feel informed, empowered, and supported throughout your pregnancy and childbirth journey.

Chapter 10: Preparing for a Cesarean Delivery

While many women hope for a vaginal delivery, sometimes a cesarean delivery, or c-section, is necessary. A c-section is a surgical procedure in which the baby is delivered through an incision made in the mother's abdomen and uterus. If you know in advance that you will be having a c-section, here are some things you can do to prepare:

1. Learn about the procedure: Talk to your healthcare provider about what to expect during the c-section. You can also watch videos or read about the procedure to help you feel more prepared.

2. Understand the risks: While c-sections are generally safe, there are risks associated with any surgery. Make sure you understand the risks and benefits of the procedure.

3. Plan for recovery: Recovery from a c-section can take longer than recovery from a vaginal delivery. Make sure you have support at home to help with tasks like lifting and caring for your baby.

4. Talk to your healthcare provider about pain management: Your healthcare provider can help you develop a plan for pain management after the c-section. This may include medication or other techniques.

5. Discuss anesthesia options: Depending on the reason for the c-section and your individual needs, you may be given a spinal block, epidural, or general anesthesia. Talk to your healthcare provider about your options and what to expect.

6. Prepare for breastfeeding: Breastfeeding after a c-section is possible, but may require some adjustments. Talk to a lactation consultant or your healthcare provider for tips on breastfeeding after a c-section.

7. Make a birth plan: While a c-section may not be the birth experience you

initially envisioned, you can still make a birth plan that reflects your preferences and goals. Discuss your preferences for pain management, breastfeeding, and skin-to-skin contact with your healthcare provider.

8. Pack a hospital bag: Be sure to pack a hospital bag that includes items you'll need for a longer hospital stay, such as comfortable clothing, toiletries, and entertainment options.

Remember that having a c-section is a common and safe way to deliver a baby when vaginal delivery is not possible. While it may not be what you hoped for, it's important to focus on the end goal: a healthy baby and a healthy you.

Chapter 11: Understanding Induction

Induction of labor is the process of artificially stimulating contractions to start labor. There are many reasons why a woman might need to be induced, including:

1. Post-term pregnancy: If a woman is past her due date and labor hasn't started naturally, her healthcare provider may recommend induction.

2. Medical conditions: Women with certain medical conditions, such as gestational diabetes or high blood

pressure, may need to be induced to avoid complications.

3. Fetal distress: If there are concerns about the baby's well-being, induction may be necessary.

4. Ruptured membranes: If a woman's water breaks and labor doesn't start on its own, induction may be necessary to avoid infection.

There are several methods of induction, including:

1. Medications: Medications such as Pitocin, a synthetic form of the hormone oxytocin, can be given to stimulate contractions.

2. Membrane stripping: This involves the healthcare provider using their finger to separate the amniotic sac from the wall of the uterus, which can stimulate contractions.

3. Breaking the water: If a woman's water hasn't broken on its own, her healthcare provider may use a tool to break the amniotic sac, which can stimulate contractions.

Some things to keep in mind when considering induction:

1. Why is induction needed? Induction may be recommended for a variety of reasons, including going past your due

date, medical complications, or concerns about the baby's health.

2. What are the risks and benefits? Induction carries some risks, including the need for additional interventions like forceps or vacuum delivery, and a higher likelihood of a c-section. However, it can also be a safe and effective way to start labor and reduce the risk of complications.

3. What are the different methods of induction? There are several methods of induction, including medication like Pitocin, mechanical methods like a Foley catheter, and natural methods like nipple stimulation. Your healthcare

provider can help you decide which method is right for you.

4. How long does it take? Induction can take several hours or even days, depending on the method used and how your body responds.

5. How will it affect my birth plan? If you have a birth plan, induction may require some adjustments. For example, you may need to change your pain management plan or be monitored more closely.

It's important to note that induction of labor can be associated with increased risks, such as a higher likelihood of c-section, so it should only be done when medically necessary. Remember that induction is a personal decision, and there is no right or wrong choice. If you are facing the possibility of induction, talk to your healthcare provider about your options and the risks and benefits of each method.

Part III: Delivery and Postpartum

Chapter 12: Delivery and Immediate Postpartum Care

Delivery is the exciting culmination of your pregnancy journey. Once labor begins, your healthcare team will guide you through the process. The delivery process can vary greatly from woman to woman, but here are some common stages:

1. Early labor: In the early stages of labor, you may experience mild contractions that gradually become stronger and more frequent.

2. Active labor: During active labor, your contractions become more intense and regular. Your cervix will dilate to 10

centimeters during this stage, which allows your baby to move through the birth canal.

3. Pushing: Once your cervix is fully dilated, you will begin to push. This can take anywhere from a few minutes to a few hours.

4. Delivery: When your baby's head emerges, your healthcare provider will guide the rest of your baby's body out of your birth canal.

After delivery, your healthcare team will monitor you and your baby closely to ensure that both of you are healthy. Here are some things you can expect during the immediate postpartum period:

1. Cord clamping: After the baby is born, the healthcare provider will clamp and cut the umbilical cord.

2. Skin-to-skin contact: Your healthcare team will encourage you to hold your baby against your bare chest for skin-to-skin contact, which has many benefits for both you and your baby.

3. Cord clamping: After the baby is born, the healthcare provider will clamp and cut the umbilical cord.

4. Breastfeeding: If you plan to breastfeed, your healthcare team can help you get started and answer any questions you may have.

5. Postpartum bleeding: It's normal to experience some bleeding and discharge after delivery. Your healthcare team can provide you with supplies and information on how to manage this.

6. Recovery: Recovery from delivery can take time, so it's important to take care of yourself in the weeks and months after giving birth.

Remember, delivery is just the beginning of your journey as a new parent. Lean on your healthcare team for support and guidance as you navigate this exciting and challenging time.

Chapter 13: Recovering from Birth

Recovering from birth can be a physical and emotional journey, and it's important to give yourself time to heal and adjust to your new role as a parent. Here are some tips to help you recover:

1. Rest: Your body needs time to recover after giving birth, so it's important to rest as much as possible. Let your friends and family help with household chores and caring for your baby so you can focus on healing.

2. Vaginal bleeding: It's normal to experience bleeding and discharge for

several weeks after delivery. Your healthcare team can provide you with supplies and information on how to manage this.

3. Pain management: It's normal to experience pain and discomfort after giving birth. Talk to your healthcare provider about pain management options, such as over-the-counter pain relievers or prescription medications.

4. Perineal care: If you had a vaginal delivery, you may experience perineal pain or swelling. Your healthcare provider can provide you with tips on perineal care, such as using a peri bottle to cleanse the area after using the restroom.

5. Nutrition: Eating a healthy diet can help support your body's recovery after birth. Focus on eating plenty of fruits, vegetables, lean protein, and whole grains.

6. Pelvic floor exercises: Pelvic floor exercises, such as Kegels, can help strengthen your pelvic muscles after birth. Your healthcare provider can provide you with guidance on how to perform these exercises.

7. Emotional support: Recovering from birth can be an emotional journey, and it's important to have a support system in place. Lean on your partner, friends, and family for emotional support, and

consider talking to a therapist if you're struggling with postpartum depression or anxiety.

8. Follow-up appointments: Your healthcare team will schedule follow-up appointments to ensure that you and your baby are healthy and recovering well.

Remember, every woman's recovery journey is unique. Be patient with yourself and give yourself time to heal and adjust to your new role as a parent.

Chapter 14: Breastfeeding and Feeding Your Newborn

Breastfeeding is a great way to provide your baby with the nutrition they need in the first few months of life. Here are some things you need to know about breastfeeding and feeding your newborn:

1. Breastfeeding basics: If you plan to breastfeed, it's important to understand the basics, including how to get a good latch, how to know if your baby is getting enough milk, and how to manage any issues that may arise.

2. Pumping and storing breastmilk: If you plan to pump breast milk, it's important

to know how to do it correctly and how to store the milk safely.

3. Bottle-feeding: If you plan to bottle-feed, it's important to choose the right type of formula and to follow the instructions carefully.

4. Feeding cues: It's important to understand your baby's feeding cues, which can include rooting, sucking on their hands, or making sucking noises.

5. Feeding schedule: In the early weeks of life, your baby may need to feed every 2-3 hours, including throughout the night. As your baby grows, they may be able to go longer between feedings.

6. Burping: After feeding, it's important to burp your baby to help them release any air they may have swallowed.

7. Breast care: It's important to care for your breasts during breastfeeding to prevent soreness and infection. Make sure you're wearing a supportive bra and keeping your nipples clean and dry.

8. Milk production: Your milk production will increase as your baby nurses. Make sure you're drinking enough fluids and getting plenty of rest to support milk production.

9. Breastfeeding positions: There are several positions you can use to breastfeed your baby, including the

cradle hold, cross-cradle hold, football hold, and side-lying position. Your healthcare team can help you find the position that works best for you and your baby.

Remember, feeding your baby is an important part of bonding and developing a close relationship with them. If you have any questions or concerns about breastfeeding or feeding your newborn, don't hesitate to reach out to your healthcare team or a lactation consultant for support and guidance.

Chapter 15: Postpartum Depression and Anxiety

Postpartum depression and anxiety are common mental health conditions that can occur after childbirth. These conditions can affect anyone, regardless of whether they had a vaginal delivery or c-section, and can be caused by a range of factors, including hormonal changes, sleep deprivation, and stress.

Here are some signs and symptoms of postpartum depression and anxiety:

- Feeling sad, hopeless, or overwhelmed
- Difficulty sleeping, even when your baby is asleep

- Loss of interest in activities you used to enjoy
- Difficulty bonding with your baby
- Feeling irritable, anxious, or on edge
- Changes in appetite or weight
- Physical symptoms, such as headaches or stomach aches
- Thoughts of self-harm or harming your baby

If you're experiencing any of these symptoms, it's important to reach out to your healthcare team right away. Postpartum depression and anxiety are treatable, and there are a range of options available, including therapy and medication.

Here are some things you can do to help prevent postpartum depression and anxiety:

1. Get enough sleep: Sleep is essential for good mental health. Try to rest whenever you can, and ask for help from friends and family if you need it.

2. Stay connected: Social support is important during the postpartum period. Stay in touch with friends and family, and consider joining a support group for new parents.

3. Take care of yourself: Self-care is important for good mental health. Take time to do things you enjoy, and don't be afraid to ask for help when you need it.

Remember, postpartum depression and anxiety are common and treatable conditions. If you're experiencing any symptoms, reach out to your healthcare team for support and guidance.

Chapter 16: Caring for Your Newborn

Caring for a newborn can be both exciting and overwhelming. Here are some tips to help you care for your new baby:

1. Feeding: As mentioned earlier, feeding your newborn is important. Whether you're breastfeeding or formula feeding, make sure your baby is fed on demand and gets enough nourishment.

2. Sleep: Newborns need a lot of sleep, but they also wake frequently. Help your baby get the sleep they need by establishing a bedtime routine and a quiet, comfortable sleep environment.

3. Diapering: Newborns go through a lot of diapers! Be sure to change your baby's diaper frequently to avoid diaper rash and irritation. Make sure to clean your baby's bottom thoroughly during diaper changes.

4. Bathing: Newborns don't need baths every day, but they do need regular cleanings. Use a gentle baby soap and warm water to clean your baby's body and scalp. Don't forget to support your baby's head and neck during bath time.

5. Bonding: Bonding with your newborn is important for both of you. Spend time holding and cuddling your baby, and talk to them often. This will help

you and your baby form a strong attachment.

6. Safety: Keeping your newborn safe is a top priority. Make sure your baby's sleep environment is safe, and never leave your baby unattended on a high surface. Also, be sure to always use a car seat when traveling with your baby.

Caring for a newborn can be a learning experience, but don't be afraid to ask for help or advice from your healthcare team, family, and friends. With a little patience and practice, you'll soon become a pro at caring for your new baby.

Chapter 17: Your New Life as a Parent

Welcoming a new baby into your life is a big adjustment, and becoming a parent is a major life change. Here are some tips to help you navigate your new life as a parent:

1. Self-Care: Taking care of yourself is important in order to be able to care for your baby. Make sure to take time for yourself to rest, relax, and recharge.

2. Adjusting to Parenthood: It's normal to feel overwhelmed, anxious, or emotional after having a baby. Give yourself time to adjust to your new role

as a parent, and don't hesitate to seek help if you're struggling.

3. Finding Support: Building a support system is key to making the transition to parenthood smoother. This can include family, friends, and support groups for new parents.

4. Balancing Work and Family: Balancing work and family can be a challenge, but it's important to find a balance that works for you and your family. Consider options like flexible work arrangements or hiring a nanny or babysitter to help.

5. Building a Routine: Establishing a routine can help you and your baby

adjust to your new life as parents. Set a schedule for feeding, sleeping, and other daily activities to help your baby feel secure and help you feel more organized.

6. Embracing Parenthood: Parenthood can be both challenging and rewarding. Embrace the joy of your new role as a parent and cherish the special moments with your baby.

Remember, every parent's experience is different, and there's no right or wrong way to navigate parenthood. Take things one day at a time, and be patient with yourself and your baby as you both learn and grow together.

Part IV: Special Considerations

Chapter 18: High-Risk Pregnancy

While most pregnancies are considered low-risk, some women may experience a high-risk pregnancy. This can be due to various factors such as age, medical conditions, or previous pregnancy complications. Here are some key points to know about a high-risk pregnancy:

1. Prenatal Care: Women with high-risk pregnancies require more frequent prenatal care to monitor their health and the health of the baby. This may include more frequent ultrasounds, blood tests, and other medical assessments.

2. Medical Management: Depending on the underlying condition or risk factor, women may require medical management such as medication or treatment to help manage the pregnancy and reduce the risk of complications.

3. Lifestyle Changes: Women with high-risk pregnancies may need to make lifestyle changes such as modifying their diet, avoiding certain activities, or reducing stress levels.

4. Birth Plan: Women with high-risk pregnancies may need to discuss their birth plan with their healthcare provider to ensure a safe delivery. This may

include a planned induction or Cesarean section.

5. Neonatal Care: Babies born to mothers with high-risk pregnancies may require specialized neonatal care after birth to monitor for any complications or health concerns.

It's important for women with high-risk pregnancies to have open communication with their healthcare provider and to follow their recommendations for prenatal care and management. By doing so, they can help ensure the best possible outcome for themselves and their baby.

Some important considerations for managing a high-risk pregnancy:

1. Consultation with a Specialist: Women with high-risk pregnancies should consider consulting with a maternal-fetal medicine specialist, who can provide specialized care and monitoring throughout the pregnancy.

2. Increased Monitoring: Women with high-risk pregnancies may require more frequent monitoring of their pregnancy, including ultrasounds, non-stress tests, and other diagnostic tests to ensure the health of the baby.

3. Managing Medical Conditions: Women with pre-existing medical conditions, such as diabetes or high blood pressure, need to manage these conditions

carefully during pregnancy, with the help of their healthcare provider.

4. Lifestyle Changes: Certain lifestyle changes can help reduce the risk of complications in high-risk pregnancies, such as avoiding alcohol, smoking, and certain medications.

5. Delivery Planning: Women with high-risk pregnancies may need to plan for a specialized delivery, such as a C-section or induction of labor, to ensure the safest possible outcome for mother and baby.

6. Emotional Support: Dealing with a high-risk pregnancy can be emotionally challenging for both the mother and her

partner. Consider seeking support from family, friends, or a therapist to help manage stress and anxiety.

While a high-risk pregnancy can be challenging, with proper care and monitoring, many women go on to have healthy pregnancies and deliveries. It's important to work closely with your healthcare provider to manage any medical conditions and ensure the best possible outcome for you and your baby.

Chapter 19: Pregnancy after 35

Pregnancy after the age of 35 is commonly referred to as "advanced maternal age." While there are some increased risks associated with pregnancy at this age, many women have successful pregnancies and healthy babies. Here are some important considerations for pregnancy after 35:

1. Fertility: Fertility declines as women age, so it may take longer to conceive. Women who are trying to conceive after 35 may want to talk to their healthcare provider about fertility testing and options.

2. Prenatal Care: Women who are pregnant after 35 may require more frequent prenatal care to monitor for potential complications, such as gestational diabetes or preeclampsia.

3. Genetic Testing: The risk of certain genetic abnormalities, such as Down syndrome, increases with maternal age. Women who are pregnant after 35 may want to consider genetic testing to assess their baby's risk.

4. Lifestyle Changes: Women who are pregnant after 35 may need to make lifestyle changes to ensure the health of their pregnancy, such as eating a healthy diet, getting regular exercise, and avoiding alcohol and tobacco.

5. Delivery Planning: Women who are pregnant after 35 may be at increased risk for certain complications during delivery, such as preterm labor or C-section delivery. It's important to discuss delivery options with your healthcare provider.

6. Emotional Support: Pregnancy after 35 can be emotionally challenging, as it may feel like there are more risks involved. Consider seeking emotional support from a therapist or support group to help manage stress and anxiety.

Pregnancy after 35 can be a healthy and successful experience with proper care and monitoring. It's important to work closely with your healthcare provider to manage any potential risks and ensure the best possible outcome for you and your baby.

Chapter 20: Pregnancy with Multiples

Pregnancy with multiples, such as twins, triplets, or more, is an exciting and challenging experience. Here are some important considerations for a pregnancy with multiples:

1. Prenatal Care: Women who are pregnant with multiples require more frequent prenatal care to monitor for potential complications, such as preterm labor, preeclampsia, or gestational diabetes.

2. Nutrition: Adequate nutrition is essential during a multiple pregnancy, as the mother is supporting the growth and development of more than one baby. Women who are pregnant with multiples may need to consume more calories and protein than women carrying a single baby.

3. Weight Gain: Women who are pregnant with multiples may need to gain more weight during pregnancy than those carrying a single baby to ensure healthy growth and development of all babies.

4. Delivery Planning: Women carrying multiples may be at increased risk for certain delivery complications, such as preterm labor or C-section delivery. It's

important to discuss delivery options with your healthcare provider.

5. Emotional Support: Pregnancy with multiples can be physically and emotionally challenging. Consider seeking emotional support from a therapist or support group to help manage stress and anxiety.

6. Preparation for Parenting Multiples: Raising multiples can be a unique and rewarding experience, but it also requires extra preparation and planning. Consider taking parenting classes specific to multiples and connecting with other parents of multiples for support and guidance.

Pregnancy with multiples requires extra care and monitoring, but with proper support and preparation, it can be a healthy and successful experience for both mother and babies. It's important to work closely with your healthcare provider to manage any potential risks and ensure the best possible outcome for you and your babies.

Chapter 21: Pregnancy Loss and Grief

Pregnancy loss, whether through miscarriage, stillbirth, or neonatal death, can be a devastating experience for parents. Here are some important considerations for navigating pregnancy loss and grief:

1. Seeking Support: It's important to seek support from loved ones, healthcare providers, and support groups. Many parents find comfort in talking to others who have experienced pregnancy loss.

2. Coping with Grief: Grief is a normal and natural response to pregnancy loss. Allow yourself to grieve in your own

way and at your own pace. Consider speaking with a therapist or grief counselor to help manage feelings of sadness, guilt, or anger.

3. Physical Recovery: Depending on the circumstances of the pregnancy loss, you may need to undergo physical recovery, such as a D&C or induction of labor. Follow your healthcare provider's instructions for self-care and recovery.

4. Planning for Future Pregnancy: If you plan to try for another pregnancy in the future, it's important to discuss any potential risks or precautions with your healthcare provider. They may recommend waiting a certain amount of

time before trying to conceive again or recommend additional testing or monitoring during a future pregnancy.

5. Honoring Your Baby: Many parents find comfort in honoring their baby's memory in some way, such as creating a memorial, planting a tree, or participating in a remembrance walk.

Navigating pregnancy loss and grief can be a difficult and painful journey, but with proper support and self-care, parents can begin to heal and move forward. It's important to take care of yourself physically and emotionally during this time and seek help when needed.

Conclusion

Congratulations on completing the happy pregnancy handbook! By now, you have learned about the various stages of pregnancy, prenatal care, labor and delivery, postpartum care, and more. Whether you are a first-time parent or a seasoned veteran, this book has provided you with valuable information and insights to help you navigate this exciting and challenging journey.

As you embark on this new chapter in your life, remember that there is no "right" way to go through pregnancy and childbirth. Every person's experience is unique and valid, and it's important to trust your instincts and listen to your body.

Remember to take care of yourself physically and emotionally during this time, and don't be afraid to seek help or support when you need it. Reach out to friends, family, or healthcare providers for guidance and support, and don't hesitate to ask questions or voice concerns.

Above all, remember that pregnancy and childbirth are incredible and transformative experiences that can bring immense joy and fulfillment. Embrace the journey, stay informed, and enjoy the ride!

Your Journey Continues: Navigating Parenthood

Now that you have completed the happy pregnancy handbook, your journey into parenthood is just beginning. Parenthood is an incredible adventure, full of ups and downs, challenges and rewards. As you move forward on this journey, here are a few things to keep in mind:

1. Trust Your Instincts: You know your child better than anyone else. Trust your instincts when it comes to making decisions about their care and well-being.

2. Prioritize Self-Care: Taking care of yourself is just as important as taking care of your child. Make time for self-care activities that help you feel relaxed, rejuvenated, and energized.

3. Seek Support: Parenthood can be overwhelming at times. Don't be afraid to ask for help or support when you need it, whether it's from a partner, family member, friend, or healthcare provider.

4. Stay Informed: As your child grows and develops, their needs will change. Stay informed about their developmental milestones and any health or safety concerns that may arise.

5. Enjoy the Journey: Parenthood can be challenging, but it's also incredibly rewarding. Enjoy the small moments and milestones, and remember to savor

the joy and wonder that comes with raising a child.

Thank you for choosing this guide to pregnancy and childbirth, and we wish you all the best as you embark on this new chapter in your life. May your journey into parenthood be filled with love, laughter, and countless happy memories.

Resources for New Parents

As a new parent, there are many resources available to you to help you navigate the joys and challenges of parenthood. Here are a few resources to consider:

1. Your Healthcare Provider: Your healthcare provider is an excellent resource for information and guidance

on your child's health and development. Don't hesitate to ask questions or voice concerns at your child's appointments.

2. Parenting Books: There are many excellent books available on various aspects of parenting, from sleep training to feeding to discipline. Look for books written by reputable authors and check reviews before making a purchase.

3. Parenting Websites and Blogs: There are countless parenting websites and blogs available, offering advice and support on various aspects of parenting. Look for websites and blogs that are reputable, informative, and up-to-date.

4. Support Groups: Joining a support group can be a great way to connect with other parents who are going through similar experiences. Look for local support groups through your healthcare provider or online.

5. Parenting Classes: Many community centers, hospitals, and healthcare providers offer parenting classes on various topics, such as childbirth education, breastfeeding, and infant care.

Remember that every child and family is unique, and what works for one family may not work for another. Trust your instincts, seek support when you need it, and enjoy this incredible journey into parenthood.

Appendix

Glossary of Pregnancy Terms

- Amniotic Fluid: The liquid that surrounds and protects the fetus in the uterus.

- Braxton Hicks Contractions: Practice contractions that occur in the uterus during pregnancy.

- Crowning: The stage of labor when the baby's head appears at the vaginal opening.

- Dilation: The opening of the cervix during labor.

- Ectopic Pregnancy: A pregnancy that occurs outside of the uterus, most commonly in the fallopian tubes.

- Fetus: The developing baby after the eighth week of pregnancy.

- Gestational Age: The age of the fetus or pregnancy, calculated from the first day of the woman's last menstrual period.

- HCG: Human Chorionic Gonadotropin, a hormone produced during pregnancy.

- Miscarriage: The loss of a pregnancy before 20 weeks.

- Placenta: The organ that develops in the uterus during pregnancy and provides oxygen and nutrients to the fetus.

- Postpartum: The period after childbirth.

- Preterm Labor: Labor that occurs before 37 weeks of pregnancy.

- Ultrasound: A diagnostic test that uses sound waves to create images of the fetus.

- Vernix: A waxy, protective substance that covers the skin of the fetus.

- Zygote: The fertilized egg before it implants in the uterus.

Helpful Websites and Organizations.
Here are some helpful websites and organizations for further information and support during pregnancy and childbirth:

1. American College of Obstetricians and Gynecologists (ACOG): ACOG is a professional organization of OB-GYNs that provides information on women's health, including pregnancy and childbirth.

2. March of Dimes: A nonprofit organization that provides education and support for moms and babies, with

a focus on preventing birth defects, premature birth, and infant mortality.

3. La Leche League International: A nonprofit organization that offers education and support for breastfeeding mothers.

4. The Bradley Method: A childbirth education program that emphasizes natural childbirth and partner-coached labor and delivery.

5. Lamaze International: A nonprofit organization that provides childbirth education and advocacy for safe and healthy birth practices.

6. Postpartum Support International: A nonprofit organization that offers support and resources for women and families experiencing postpartum depression and other perinatal mood and anxiety disorders.

7. What to Expect: A website and app that provides information and support for pregnancy and parenting, including a due date calculator, pregnancy tracker, and community forums.

8. BabyCenter: A website and app that offers information and resources for pregnancy and parenting, including a due date calculator, baby name finder, and community forums.

9. HealthyChildren.org: A website from the American Academy of Pediatrics that provides information on child health and development, including pregnancy and childbirth.